HEART HEALTHY COOKBOOK

For Women over 60

60 Days Guides on Heart-Healthy Recipes

ALAN BROOKE

TABLE OF CONTENT

INTRODUCTION

Introduction to Heart Health
for Women Over 60

Every person should be concerned about their heart health, but as women get older—especially around the age of 60—this concern becomes more perplexing. A woman's body experiences a variety of changes at this stage of life, including hormonal differences and an increased risk of developing specific medical diseases.

Risk Factors

Numerous factors increase the risk of having heart disease in women over 60. A history of diabetes, smoking, obesity, high blood pressure, high cholesterol, heart disease, and a sedentary lifestyle are a few examples. It's crucial to be aware of these risk factors and to maintain proactive control over them.

Adjustments to Hormones

After menopause, women's estrogen levels decrease, which may be detrimental to heart health. Because estrogen is thought to protect blood vessels, its absence may increase the risk of heart disease. Understanding how hormones affect heart health is crucial to conclude hormone replacement therapy, if necessary.

Symptoms:

Women may experience a variety of heart disease symptoms in contrast to men. Women may have minor aches or boredom as normal aging symptoms. Disadvantages, breathing difficulties, chest pain, and discomfort in the jaw, neck, or upper back are a few examples of these symptoms. To evaluate and resolve problems as soon as possible, it's critical to be aware of these warning indicators.

Preventive measures

Heart health can be promoted in women over 60 in several ways. Among these are reducing trans and saturated fats and maintaining a balanced diet rich in fruits, vegetables, whole grains, and lean proteins. Regular physical activity and weight control are more crucial. Furthermore, quitting smoking and using stress-reduction techniques can significantly reduce the risk of developing heart disease.

Regular Checkups:

Regular doctor visits are required to monitor heart health. Routine blood pressure checks, cholesterol tests, and discussions with medical specialists about your heart disease risk factors are all essential to early intervention and prevention of heart disease.

Medications and Treatment:

Periodically using medications or medical methods may be necessary to properly control heart health. Women over 60 should carefully discuss their treatment options with their doctors to choose the best course of action, which may involve prescription medication, lifestyle change, or, in more serious scenarios, surgical procedures.

Assistance and Guidance:

It may be created so that people can join charities or find out more about heart health for women over 60. A terrific method to learn is to discuss ideas and offer fervent encouragement to others going through similar struggles.

Heart health is a crucial component of overall well-being for women over 60. By being aware of the risks and other factors that occur during this stage of life and adopting preventative measures to maintain their hearts in reasonable form, women can lead meaningful lives that are heart-healthy well into their senior years. It's never too late to make positive changes that could lead to a longer, more nutrient-dense life and prioritize heart health.

CHAPTER ONE

Understanding Heart Health

Understanding heart health is crucial for women over 60 because it continues to be the leading cause of mortality in this demographic. Here is a detailed summary:

Factors at Risk for Heart Disease

Age:

Age increases the risk of heart disease in women, especially after menopause.

Family History

A history of heart disease in the

family can increase risk.

Menopause:

Estrogen levels decrease after menopause, increasing the risk of heart disease.

Lifestyle Factors

Significant risk factors include smoking, eating poorly, living a sedentary lifestyle, being overweight, and using excessive amounts of alcohol.

Symptoms:

Fatigue, shortness of breath, nausea, or discomfort in the jaw, neck, or back are common indicators that a woman may have heart disease.

It's important to identify these small symptoms as potential heart issues.

Screening and diagnosis

Regular check-ups are required to monitor blood pressure, cholesterol, and blood sugar levels. Testing procedures such as pressure tests, echocardiograms, and coronary angiography might be necessary for the diagnosis.

Prevention:

Diet:

Lowering the risk requires eating a heart-healthy diet low in sodium and saturated fats and abundant in fruits, vegetables, whole grains, and lean proteins.

Exercise:

Regular exercise, like brisk walking or swimming, is beneficial.

Maintaining Heart Health.

Weight Management:

Maintaining a healthy weight lowers the risk of developing heart disease.

Stop Smoking:

Quitting smoking is one of the most important things you can do if you smoke.

Alcohol Restrictions:

The key is moderation; have no more than one drink each day.

Reduced Stress:

Yoga and meditation are examples of anxiety-reduction techniques that can benefit heart health.

Medical Care and Medication:

Drugs for blood pressure or statins (which lower cholesterol) may be prescribed while taking into account a person's personal risk factors.
In dire cases, procedures like angioplasty or coronary artery bypass surgery may be required.

Understanding Differences in Gender

Women could display a wider range of symptoms than men, and they might react to therapy differently. Healthcare providers should consider these gender-specific issues.

regular assessments

Regular exams with a medical practitioner can identify issues early and permit quick action.

Auxiliary System

Having a strong support system and discussing issues with family and friends can help reduce anxiety.

Mental Health:

Situations involving mental health, such as melancholy or worry, must be managed because they may have an impact on heart health.

Alterations in Lifestyle:

By encouraging a healthy lifestyle for the entire family, the risk of heart disease can be reduced overall.

Understanding heart health for women at 60 involves recognizing risk factors, being aware of notable signs, adopting a heart-healthy lifestyle, and maintaining a routine of medical tests. To reduce the risk of heart disease in this population, proactive healthcare choices and education are crucial.

CHAPTER TWO

Benefits of Eating Balanced

To maintain their health and well-being throughout this stage of life, women over 60 must keep a balanced diet. Here, we look in depth at the significance of a balanced diet for women of this age group:

Necessary Nutrients

Women over 60 have different nutrient demands, as was mentioned in the section about persons. To support overall vitality and maintain bone health, they must consume enough essential nutrients like calcium, vitamin D, vitamin B12, and iron.

Bone Health:

As we age, osteoporosis becomes a bigger problem, therefore it's critical to preserve healthy bones and reduce the risk of fractures with a balanced diet rich in calcium and vitamin D.

Heart Health:

Heart disease risk rises with age. You can lower your risk of heart-related issues by maintaining healthy blood pressure and cholesterol levels with a balanced diet reduced in sodium, cholesterol, saturated fats, and trans fats.

Weight Management:

Maintaining a healthy weight is crucial for women over 60 who want to avoid conditions like diabetes, heart disease, and arthritis. Weight management can be aided by a well-balanced diet that provides the necessary nutrients while limiting calorie intake.

Internal Wellness

As we grow older, digestive issues could arise. A diet high in fiber from fruits, vegetables, whole grains, and legumes can help you manage constipation.

Mental Stamina:

Eating nutritiously can support cognitive enactment. Fruits and vegetables, leafy greens, and fish with omega-3 fatty acids are a few foods that are rich in antioxidants and can prevent cognitive decline.

System of Defense:

As the immune system deteriorates with age, a nutritious diet high in vitamins, minerals, and antioxidants can support the immune system and reduce the risk of infections and illness.

Hormonal Balance:

Hormone problems emerge in menopausal or postmenopausal

women. A select few nutrients, such as the phytoestrogens found in soy products, may help lessen menopause symptoms.

Maintaining Muscular Mass

One well-known side effect of aging is muscle loss. Combining resistance training with a diet rich in protein will help you keep your muscles stable and strong.

Excellent Mental Health

A balanced diet can support improved mental health and emotional stability. Foods high in complex carbohydrates can help control blood sugar levels, reducing mood swings.

Managing Chronic Illnesses:

Eating a diet high in fruits, vegetables, whole grains, and lean meats can lower the chance of developing chronic diseases like diabetes, some types of cancer, and hypertension.

Life Expectancy:

In the end, women over 60 who ate a balanced diet had a higher overall quality of life. It stores the food and energy required to continue being independent, active, and engaged in daily activities.

Women over 60 must consume a balanced diet tailored to their unique nutritional needs to remain healthy, vital, and long-lived. A licensed dietitian or healthcare expert can help you create a personalized dietary plan that considers your health objectives and concerns at this stage of life.

CHAPTER THREE

How to Build a Filling, Healthful Pantry

It's crucial to have a robust and nutritious pantry if you want to keep a balanced diet and make sure you always have sustaining options available. With the aid of a well-stocked pantry, you can plan healthful meals even when you are short on time or fresh supplies. Here is a detailed tutorial on building a potent, nourishing pantry:

Establish Your Needs

Before you start, consider your food selections and any dietary limitations. Consider any special food restrictions you have, such as vegetarianism, veganism, or gluten intolerance. Using this, you can modify your pantry to suit your requirements.

Choose Whole Grains:

Whole grains are a necessity for a balanced pantry. Choose items made from whole grains, such as brown rice, quinoa, whole wheat pasta, oats, and cereal. These provide complex carbs, essential minerals, and fiber.

Build Up Your Legumes:

Beans, lentils, and chickpeas are excellent sources of plant-based fiber and protein. They can be included in a variety of foods, such as soups, stews, salads, and more.

When to Use Canned Tomatoes:

Canned tomatoes are a flexible component that can be used to make sauces, soups, and stews. Choose foods that haven't been salted or sweetened.

Select Healthful Oils:

Good choices for salad dressing and reading include coconut oil, avocado oil, and olive oil. They provide readily available heart-healthy fats.

Don't forget the canned fish:

Salmon, tuna, and sardines in cans are excellent sources of protein and omega-3 fatty acids. Additionally helpful for preparing salad dressing and sandwiches.

Ample Herbs and Spices to Purchase:

Herbs and spices can enhance flavor without adding too much fat or salt. Typical options include paprika, cinnamon, cumin, cinnamon, oregano, and basil.

Must Include Nuts and Seeds:

Almonds, walnuts, chia seeds, and flaxseeds are rich sources of fiber, healthy fats, and protein. They make the perfect snack or topping for yogurt and oat bran.

Maintain a Variety of Canned Vegetables:

When fresh options aren't available, using canned vegetables like corn, peas, and green beans in dishes is simple. Pick low-sodium substitutes.

Store healthy snacks:

Stock your cabinet with healthy snacks like popcorn, whole-grain crackers, and dried fruits to satiate cravings.

Cleverly sweeten:

If you need a sweetener, think about substituting stevia, honey, or maple syrup for refined sugar.

Maintain a Selection of Whole-Grain Flours:

Keep whole-grain flour on hand if baking is your preferred method of cooking.

Make plans for specialty items:

Depending on your dietary restrictions, you could require items like gluten-free pasta, almond butter, or nutritional yeast. Make certain you have access to these.

Trading Stock

Keep an eye on dates of expiration and rotate your pantry products to prevent food from going bad.

Ensure order:

Spend money on shelves and storage containers to keep your pantry orderly. Label containers so that ingredients can be found immediately.

Think About Your Portion Size

While having a well-stocked pantry is important, you should attempt to limit the amount of food you buy that you won't use frequently.

Organize Meals Using

Include cupboard essentials whenever you plan your weekly meals to make cooking more practical and cost-effective.

A robust, healthy pantry requires time to build. To cook wholesome and delectable meals, regularly check the contents of your pantry, resupply as necessary, and continue experimenting with new products and recipes.

CHAPTER FOUR

Including whole grains and fiber

By integrating whole grains and fiber into your diet, you can significantly improve your health and sense of well-being. Whole grains and fiber have many other benefits besides aiding in digestion and reducing the incidence of chronic diseases. Detailed information on why and how to include them in your diet is provided below:

Why Whole Grains and Fiber Are Important:

Nutrient-Rich:

Whole grains are a great source of important nutrients such as vitamins, minerals, and antioxidants. Whole grains and other plant-based diets contain fiber, which is essential for overall health.

Internal Wellness

Fiber adds weight to your diet, promotes regular bowel motions, and guards against constipation. It can also help with the treatment of conditions like IBS.

Blood Sugar Control:

Whole grains' slow glucose absorption aids in blood sugar regulation. The most likely beneficiaries of this might be diabetics.

Heart Health:

A diet rich in whole grains and fiber is associated with a lower risk of heart disease. It helps maintain normal blood pressure and reduces cholesterol.

Weight Management:

You feel full after eating foods high in fiber, which may motivate you to eat fewer calories and maintain a healthier weight.

Cancer Risk is Lower

A diet high in fiber may lower your risk of getting several malignancies, particularly colon cancer, according to multiple studies.

Including whole grains and fiber in your diet:

Choose Whole Grains:

Choose whole grains over processed grains wherever possible. Whole grains include things like whole wheat, brown rice, quinoa, oats, and barley, to name a few. In these grains, the entire fiber- and mineral-rich kernel is preserved.

Check Labels:

Before making a packaged food purchase, look at the ingredient list. Look for grains that say "whole" in front of them. Better choices include "whole wheat flour" or "whole oats."

Start your Day Off Right:

Eat a breakfast that is heavy in fiber to get your day started right. Oatmeal, whole-grain cereal, and whole-grain toast with peanut butter are all excellent choices.

Boosting Meal Volume:

Whole grains should be a part of both lunch and dinner. Use whole wheat pasta instead of regular pasta, brown rice in place of white rice, and quinoa as a side dish.

Smart Snacking:

At mealtimes, choose foods that are high in fiber. Whole-grain crackers with hummus, fruit, almonds, and pistachios are all fantastic substitutes.

Vegetables and legumes

Include vegetables and legumes in your diet as they are great providers of fiber. Consider serving lentil soup, bean salads, or roasted veggies as a side dish.

Gradual Transition:

If it isn't already a part of your diet, add fiber gradually to prevent digestive discomfort. Bloating and gas could result from an increase in fiber consumption that is too quick.

Stay hydrated

When consuming extra fiber, make sure to drink plenty of water. Because fiber may absorb water, your digestive system can work more effectively.

Remember that gaining the benefits of whole grains and fiber requires a balanced diet. In addition to these dietary changes, maintaining an active lifestyle and limiting portion sizes can improve general health. Consult with a healthcare professional or nutritionist for assistance on how to incorporate whole grains and fiber into your diet if you have any specific dietary restrictions or health problems.

CHAPTER FIVE

Proteins for Optimal Cardiovascular Health

To reduce their chance of developing heart disease, women over 60 must maintain their cardiovascular health at its highest level. Understanding how proteins help to maintain cardiovascular health is essential. What information about proteins can women over 60 learn to improve their cardiovascular health? An extensive summary is provided below:

For Women Over 60, Cardiovascular Health Is Important:

Cardiovascular disease, which includes heart disease and stroke, is one of the leading causes of death in women over the age of 60. As a woman matures, hormonal changes and lifestyle choices may increase her chance of developing heart-related issues. Therefore, it's imperative to prioritize cardiovascular health through a variety of methods, including diet.

Contribution of Proteins to Cardiovascular Health

Protein is one of the most crucial macronutrients for promoting cardiovascular health. They aid heart health in several ways:

Control of blood pressure:

Various proteins can control blood pressure. Angiotensin-converting enzyme (ACE) inhibitors, for instance, are a class of medications that reduce blood pressure while easing the strain on the heart.

Cholesterol Balance:

Proteins regulate cholesterol levels, which is crucial for cardiovascular health. Certain proteins raise the "good" cholesterol known as high-density lipoprotein (HDL), which reduces the risk of arterial plaque development.

Prevention of Inflammation

The risk of heart disease is increased by ongoing inflammation. Certain proteins contain anti-inflammatory properties that can help to lessen inflammation in the cardiovascular system.

Different Protein Sources

Focusing on getting enough protein from a variety of sources is important for women over 60. These include:

Healthy Meats

Fish, skinless poultry, and lean meats like cattle and pigs are all fantastic sources of high-quality protein.

Plant-based proteins:

Legumes, nuts, seeds, and tofu are sources of protein in addition to providing heart-healthy elements including fiber and unsaturated fats.

dairy products

Low-fat or fat-free dairy products are strong in protein and can be a part of a heart-healthy diet.

Whole Grains:

Whole grains high in protein, such as quinoa and brown rice, are crucial parts of a diet that supports heart health.

Optimal Nutrition for Cardiovascular Health

Women over 60 should aim for a well-balanced diet with a variety of nutrients to maintain heart health. This should include:

Fruits and vegetables:

These fiber- and antioxidant-rich meals help to improve overall cardiovascular health by lowering inflammation.

Recommended Fats:

Eat foods high in unsaturated fat like avocados, olive oil, and fatty fish as part of your diet.

Speak with a Medical Expert

A certified dietitian or healthcare provider should be consulted by women over 60 for specific advice on protein intake and cardiovascular health. They could assess the individual's health needs and provide tailored guidance.

Understanding how proteins contribute to maintaining cardiovascular health is crucial for women over 60. A balanced diet rich in high-quality protein sources can significantly reduce the risk of heart disease and increase general well-being when combined with other heart-healthy lifestyle choices. Always consult a healthcare professional for individualized guidance determined by a person's health situation and goals.

CHAPTER SIX

Fruits and Veggies that are Heart-Friendly

Heart-friendly fruits and vegetables are essential for women over 60 as they offer a wealth of health benefits that can help preserve cardiovascular health and general well-being. The following information summarizes the potency of various foods for this particular age group:

Antioxidants in Great Supply:

Vitamins C and E, two antioxidants included in fruits and vegetables, aid in the battle against free radicals and reduce oxidative stress. Because oxidative stress has been connected to heart disease and other aging-related health issues, women over 60 should pay particular attention to this.

dietary fiber

Numerous fruits and vegetables contain high levels of dietary fiber. Fiber helps people maintain heart health and prevent disorders like diabetes and obesity by promoting good digestion, lowering blood sugar levels, and assisting with weight management.

little salt:

Heart-healthy fruits and vegetables naturally contain minimal levels of sodium. A low-sodium diet is essential for older people because it lowers blood pressure and lowers the risk of heart disease.

Potassium-Rich:

Bananas, oranges, and spinach are all high in potassium, a mineral that lowers blood pressure. Controlling blood pressure is crucial for heart health, particularly as women get older.

Lower Stroke Risk:

Eating a variety of fruits and vegetables has been related to a lower risk of stroke. The risk of stroke tends to increase with age, therefore this is crucial for women over 60.

Foods Good for the Heart

Several fruits and vegetables have particular nutrients that are very beneficial for heart health. While leafy greens like kale and spinach include vitamin K, which aids in blood clotting, citrus fruits contain flavonoids, which have been linked to enhanced heart health.

Effects on Cholesterol Reduction

Several fruits and vegetables, including oats, apples, and eggplants, can lower cholesterol.

One can reduce the danger of heart disease and control the levels of cholesterol by eating these meals.

Weight Management:

For the health of your heart, you must maintain a healthy weight. Since they are low in calories and high in nutrients, vegetables, and fruits are a fantastic alternative for weight management. They can assist senior ladies in cutting calories without sacrificing essential nutrients.

Better control of blood sugar

Diabetes is more prevalent as people age. Some fruits and vegetables, such as berries and broccoli, can help control blood sugar levels because of their low glycemic index. For controlling and avoiding diabetes, this is crucial.

overall wellbeing

A diet rich in fruits and vegetables supports not only overall health but also heart health. For women over 60 to lead active, fulfilling lives, they need to have more energy, have better cognitive function, and have healthier skin.

Fruits and vegetables are the cornerstone of a heart-healthy diet for women over 60. By consuming a range of these foods in their regular meals, they can significantly reduce their risk of developing heart disease, stroke, and other age-related health issues, which will also enhance their general well-being. It is essential to see a nutritionist or healthcare professional to create a personalized diet plan that suits each person's needs and preferences.

CHAPTER SEVEN

Techniques for Heart-Healthy Cooking

Cooking techniques for heart health must be used to maintain cardiovascular health. These strategies place a strong emphasis on reducing bad fat intake, reducing salt consumption, and increasing intake of heart-healthy nutrients including nutrients such as fiber, and omega-3 fatty acids. Here is a detailed breakdown:

Grilling and Roasting

Grilling and broiling are the best cooking methods for heart health. By enabling additional fat to flow away from the food, they lower the total calorie and saturated fat content of the food. Lean cuts of meat, poultry, or fish can be marinated with herbs and spices in place of oil-based marinades.

Steaming:

The heart-healthy method of steaming preserves the natural flavors and minerals of food. Because it doesn't require additional fats, it goes nicely with vegetables, fish, and poultry. Additionally, steaming helps preserve the food's flavor and appearance.

Baking and roasting

The heart-protective cooking techniques of baking and roasting use the oven's dry heat. You can roast veggies, chicken, or fish with a little extra fat. To allow the excess fat from meats to drain, use a baking rack.

Stir-Frying:

Stir-frying is a fast and heart-healthy preparation technique. Make sure to include a lot of vegetables, lean proteins, flavorful spices and herbs, a tiny quantity of heart-healthy oils like olive or canola, and other ingredients. Stay away from heavy, salty sauces.

Poaching:

Poaching involves cooking food gently in a liquid, most typically water or a flavorful broth. Fish, poultry, and fruits can all be prepared using this low-fat method. Poached foods retain their flavor and moisture without adding additional calories.

Regarding Vapor:

By being sealed with a vacuum and heated to a set temperature in a water bath, food is cooked sous vide. This method seals in the flavors and nutrients without the need for extra lipids. But it does require specialist equipment.

Inefficient Cooking

With a slow cooker, making heart-healthy meals is simple. Nutrient-dense stews, soups, and pies can be made with lean meats, beans, and lots of vegetables. Being ready with a heart-healthy dinner when you get home is a useful strategy.

Microwaving:

Particularly vegetables, heart-healthy meals can be swiftly and simply made in the microwave. Utilize microwave-safe containers, a small amount of water, and a cover to steam vegetables without using additional oil.

Herbs and spices:

To enhance flavor without introducing salt or unhealthy fats, experiment with a wide range of herbs and spices. They can transform a simple recipe into a delectable, heart-healthy dinner.

Controlling Portions

Whatever the cooking technique, portion control is essential for heart health. Stay away from heavy meals.

I Utilize heart-healthy fats:

When you need to eat fats, pick heart-healthy fats like oil derived from olives, can, or avocado oil. Unsaturated and polyunsaturated fatty acids, which are abundant in these lipids may benefit heart health.

Limit your consumption of sodium:

Salt consumption needs to be reduced for optimal heart function. Use herbs, spices, and salt substitutes to flavor your food instead of using excessive amounts of salt.

Remember that choosing the right ingredients is just as crucial to a heart-healthy diet as using the right cooking techniques. Increase the amount of whole grains, lean meats, fresh veggies, and grains in their entirety in your diet. Consult a competent dietician or member of the healthcare team for personalized guidance on keeping a heart-healthy diet tailored to your unique needs.

CHAPTER EIGHT

Heart-healthy breakfast

A heart-healthy breakfast is crucial for women over 60 since it can help control a range of cardiovascular risk indicators that become more prevalent as we get older. A balanced breakfast can promote heart health by helping you to keep your weight, cholesterol, and blood pressure under control. A complete approach to making a heart-healthy breakfast for women over 60 can be found below:

Foods High in Fiber:

Begin your day with foods high in fiber, e pancakes or whole-grain breads. The potential of soluble fiber to lower levels of bad cholesterol, also known as LDL, lowers the risk of heart disease.

Berries:

Use a range of berries, such as berries, blueberries, and raspberries. They are rich in antioxidants, fiber, and nutrients that support heart health and reduce stress.

Nuts and Seeds:

Your morning meal should include some unprocessed nuts or seeds like almonds, walnuts, or chia seeds, for instance. They provide fiber, healthy fats, and sterols from plants that can lower cholesterol.

Low-fat dairy items or dairy alternatives:

Almond or milk are dairy-free options, or go for low-fat yogurt or milk. These provide calcium and protein instead of the amount of saturated fat found in whole milk.

Healthy Protein

Use tofu, lean turkey or chicken sausages, and eggs (preferably boiled or cooked) as lean protein sources. Protein keeps the muscle groups healthy and gives you a feeling of fullness.

Fruits:

Incorporate berries with other heart-healthy foods like oranges, apples, and bananas. They deliver vital vitamins and minerals while being low in salt and saturated fats.

Unruly Fish

Consider having fatty fish for breakfast a few times a week, like mackerel or salmon. This fish has a lot of omega-3 fatty acids, among others, which may help reduce the risk of heart disease.

Whole Grains:

Toast or whole-grain bread should be used in place of white bread. Whole grains provide more minerals, vitamins, and fiber, all of which help to improve heart wellness.

Controlling Portions

Pay attention to portion sizes. Weight gain can occur even when eating nourishing meals in excess, which raises the risk of heart disease.

Reduce additional sugar intake:

Limit your consumption of sugary cereals, pastries, and drinks. Excessive consumption of sugar increases your risk of creating weight gain and heart disease.

Hydration:

Start your day with a glass of water or herbal tea to stay hydrated. Drinking enough water is essential for overall health in addition to assisting with appetite control.

Mindful Eating:

Take your time enjoying and fully chewing your breakfast. Eating with awareness can improve digestion and reduce overeating.

Cowell-being nutritionist

If you have certain dietary restrictions or health concerns, think about visiting with a qualified dietician or nutritionist. They can provide you with specialized guidance that is tailored to your requirements.

A heart-friendly meal is simply a small part of a bigger healthy lifestyle, so remember that at all times. In addition to giving up smoking, sustaining heart health in older women calls for regular exercise, stress reduction, and a good diet. Always get specific advice from a medical practitioner about how to manage your cardiovascular risk factors.

CHAPTER NINE

Nutrition-Packed Lunches

Nutrient-dense meals are crucial for women over 60 to support their general health and well-being. As we age, our nutritional requirements change, making it even more important to eat a balanced diet rich in essential nutrients. Here is a comprehensive guide to creating nutrient-dense meals tailored to the needs of women over 60:

Lite Protein

A reliable supply of healthy protein ought to be part of your diet. Fish (such as salmon or tuna) is a great option, as are subjected to chicken, turkey, tofu, lentils, and other meats. Protein is essential for maintaining physiological function, bone health, and muscle mass.

High-fiber greens

Make sure your lunch has a range of vibrant vegetables to ensure you get a balanced intake of vitamins and minerals. Broccoli, carrots, bell peppers, and leafy greens are your best bets. Fiber improves digestion, reduces blood sugar, and promotes heart health.

Appropriate Fats:

Healthy fat options for your meal should include avocados, nuts, seeds, and olive oil. These fats help boost brain function, keep joints in good condition, and reduce the risk of acquiring chronic diseases like heart disease.

Whole Grains:

Instead, choose whole grains like brown rice, quinoa, whole wheat bread, or spaghetti made with whole grains. These provide fiber, enduring energy, and essential nutrients like B vitamins.

substitutes for dairy products

Include dairy products like yogurt or cheese (choose low-fat or non-fat variants if you'd like) or dairy-free alternatives like almond milk or soy yogurt to ensure proper calcium consumption for bone health.

Hydration:

To stay hydrated during the day, consume lots of water, green tea, or reduced fruit juices. Proper hydration is crucial for healthy skin, digestion, and bodily functions in general.

Fruit:

Serve some fresh fruit to yourself for dinner or a side dish. Vitamins and antioxidants are abundant in apples, berries, and citrus fruits. They can help keep the immune system and skin healthy.

Controlling Portions

Keep an eye on your portion sizes to avoid overeating. Because digestion usually slows down as we age, managing your portions can help you achieve a healthy weight.

Consume less processed food:

Limit the use of refined foods, which are often high in salt, sugar, and unhealthy fats. These may contribute to several health issues, including obesity and hypertension.

Particular Considerations

If you are experiencing specific dietary restrictions or medical conditions, speak with a licensed nutritionist or another medical professional to personalize your lunch alternatives.

Variety:

To get a range of nutrients over time, switch up your lunch choices. Providing a larger variety of vitamins and minerals can also lessen dietary monotony.

Prepare meals:

Prepare your lunches in advance to ensure that they meet your dietary demands. This may help you avoid grabbing unhealthy foods when you're hurried and hungry.

To get individualized advice based on your health problems and dietary preferences, speak with a healthcare practitioner or registered dietitian. Keep in mind that everyone has different nutritional needs. Maintaining a balanced diet is crucial for aging gracefully and being active and energetic into old life. Nutrient-rich meals are one aspect of eating well.